THE UNIQUE KINESIOLOGY TAPING HAND BOOK

YOUR EFFECTIVE PRACTICAL GUIDE FOR DAILY LIFESTYLE, FITNESS, SPORTS, INJURY PREVENTION AND OVERCOMING STRAINS

DOCTOR DAVID TAYLOR

TABLE OF CONTENT

CHAPTER 1

INTRODUCTION
WHAT IS KINESIOLOGY

Kinesiology categorically came from the Greek words for the study of movement. It evaluates health by exploring the training program from muscles. The most principle of applied physiology includes: A stress that strains the complete body could manifest objectively as a weakening of one muscle.

Kinesiology visualizes muscles as coupled to specific organs, and it uses manual muscle testing to gauge the health of the patient. Whereas typical drugs uses muscle testing as a way of assessing the structural and purposeful health of the fiber bundle unit, applied physiology makes use of this method to grasp organ-related, biological process or emotional imbalances within the body.

This testing employs the strength or weakness of a muscle to urge data concerning the organ that it's coupled to, and also the demand of the body for a selected nutrient. The muscle testing utilized is by holding the muscle in isometric contraction against a resistance applied outwardly, instead of voluntary contraction against associate unmovable object. This is often known as Kendall's technique. Provocative tests square measure used alongside muscle testing.

This form of manual muscle testing therefore identifies the matter, whether or not within the physical (in relevance the nervous, muscular or skeletal system), emotional or organic chemistry (metabolic) realm, still as within the mental, non-organic sphere, with un-wellness that isn't arising or associated with the symptomatic systems. Practitioners of applied physiology claim to market physical, emotional, mental and non secular health by distinguishing and treating these issues.

Kinesiologists attempt to work with and utilize the healing powers, or life forces, of the body itself. They draw support from Chinese treatment still as from chiropractics. It's additionally part based mostly upon applied physiology, that measures muscle strength. It's so not based mostly upon the Western model of medication, visualizing the body rather as associate energy system.

CHAPTER 2

UNDERSTANDING THE JOB OF A KINESIOLOGIST

The basic premise of physiology is that the body has its own healing energy and is doing its best to worry for itself, however typically wants a bit facilitate to realize this state. Physiology, therefore, is also understood as a system of natural health care which mixes muscle observance with the principles of Chinese drugs to assess energy and body perform. The kinesiologist allows this method by applying a spread of light however powerful healing techniques to boost health, well-being and vitality.

Kinesiologists faucet into energies that different modalities don't assess. They appear on the far side the symptoms, and don't diagnose or treat named diseases. In fact, they are doing not limit themselves to handling ailments, since energy equalization will bring an individual nearer to achieving any goal of their selection, whether or not in sport, relationships, learning or handling life normally. They involved with imbalances within the body's energy, and during this respect, have shut links with the stylostixis construct of energy flow. A kinesiologist acknowledges that there are a unit flows of energy among the body that relate not solely to the muscles however to each tissue and organ that move to build the body a living, feeling being.

Kinesiologists apply muscle testing to spot and proper energy blockages among the body; it's a natural feedback system that receives data via nerve pathways and therefore the meridian system of the brain and body. This muscle feedback system provides instant access into the holistic data command by the subconscious brain. A weak muscle take a look at will so be associate indicator that stress has a tellingly negative impact somewhere within the system. By accessing the bio-system via this muscle observance tool, kinesiologists will get quite specific and really quickly come back up with the proper answers.

Duties of a kinesiologist that is as listed:

Help people deal with physical injuries'

Apply varied healing techniques so as to alleviate muscle ailments

Work to manage, rehabilitate, and stop disorders that impede movement

Monitor patients to make sure their program produces the specified effects

Demonstrate correct muscle movement so as to forestall injuries

May work to boost motor learning skills in patients littered with brain disease, autism, and different motor and medicine issues

May promote engineering science geographic point body postures and instrumentality choice

CHAPTER 3

HOW KINESIOLOGY WORKS DOES TAPE

Kinesiology tape is indeed very stretchy.

Kinesio tape was created with a proprietary mix of cotton and nylon. It's designed to mimic the skin's snap thus you'll be able to use your full vary of motion. The tape's medical-grade adhesive is additionally waterproof and robust enough to remain on for

3 to 5 days, even whereas you're employed out or take showers.

When the tape is gently applied on your body, it thereby recoils slightly, gently lifting your skin. It's so believed that this helps to forms a microscopic house between your skin and therefore the tissues beneath it.

CHAPTER 4

WHAT KINESIOLOGY TAPE IS USED FOR

For Treating Injuries:

Physical therapists typically use physiology tape jointly a part of Associate in nursing overall treatment arrange for folks who've been gashed. The yank medical care, physiotherapy, physiatrists, therapy reports that physiology tape is best once it's utilized in conjunction with alternative treatments like manual therapy.

"We use physiology tape to mitigate pain and swelling," Schooled says, "but it's forever used as Associate in nursing adjunct to what we're making an attempt to accomplish."

For enhancing performance:

Some athletes use physiology tape recordings to assist them attain peak performance and defend against injury once they're competitor in special events.

"A ton of runners use this tape whenever they run a marathon," Schooled says. "We typically place the tape on the striated muscle as some way of 'waking up' the muscle and reminding it to stay operating."

For Managing scars:

Although you ought to ne'er use physiology tape on associate open wound, there's some scientific proof to counsel that physiology tape will improve the long look of scars when surgery or injury. This is often undoubtedly a treatment you ought to sit down with a doctor firstly.

For supporting weak zones:

Kinesiology tape is additionally wont to add additional support to muscles or joints that require it. If you have got stress syndrome, band fiction, or mythical being redness, physiology tape recording may assist you.

Unlike white medical or athletic tape, physiology tape enables you to move unremarkably. In fact, some studies show that it will enhance movement and endurance. Studies on athletes have shown that once physiology tape is employed on worn out muscles, performance improves.

CHAPTER 5

HOW TO APPLY KINESIOLOGY TAPE

You should forever check with a therapist WHO is trained within the correct application of physiology tape before you are trying to place it on yourself.

A therapist can show you ways to use the tape within the pattern that may facilitate your specific downside. Tape is applied in AN X, Y, I, or fan pattern, counting on your goals.

You'll additionally want each stabilization and decompression strips.

Your therapist will watch you follow applying and removing the tape before you are trying it reception.

"Taping isn't a permanent resolution," Schooled says. "You wish to make your strength and ability, as a result of correcting the basis downside is essential."

To apply this tape in good ways, kindly remember the following few steps as stated:

Clean and dry the realm 1st. Lotions and oils will forestall the tape from sticking out.

Trim excess hair. Fine hair shouldn't be a drag; however dense hair may keep the tape from obtaining a decent grip on your skin.

For many treatments, you'll begin by tearing the backing paper within the center.

Cut rounded corners at the ends of every stripe if they don't have already had them. The rounded corners area unit less possible to induce snagged against clothing; and helps to stay the tape on longer.

 Once you apply the primary tab to anchor the strip, let the top recoil slightly when you are taking off the backing paper. You don't wish any stretch within the last 2 inches at either finish, as a result of those tabs area unit simply to carry the tape in situ. If you stretch the ends, the tape can pull your skin, that may cause irritation or build the tape detach sooner.

 Keep your fingers on the packing paper to carry the tape. Touching the adhesive half can build it less sticky.

Your expert will allow you to knowledge a lot of stretch to use within the treatment space. To induce a seventy five % stretch, extend the tape as way because it can go then unleash it a few quarter of its length.

Once you stretch the tape, use the total length of your thumb across the tape to induce a fair stretch.

When you apply the tape, rub the strip smartly for many

seconds. Heat activates the glue. Full adhesion typically takes around twenty minutes.

CHAPTER 6

WHEN YOU SHOULD NOT USE KINESIOLOGY TAPE

There are some circumstances within which physiology tape shouldn't be used. They embrace the subsequent.

Open wounds: Exploitation tape over a wound may lead to infection or skin harm.

Deep vein occlusion: Increasing fluid flow might cause a blood to dislodge, which could be fatal.

Active cancer: Increasing blood provide to a cancerous growth may be dangerous.

Lymphoid tissue removal: Increasing fluid wherever a node is missing might cause swelling.

Diabetes: If you've got reduced sensation in some areas, you would possibly not notice a reaction to the tape.

Allergy: If your skin is sensitive to adhesives, you'll trigger a robust reaction.

Fragile skin: If your skin is vulnerable to tearing, you ought to avoid putting tape on that.

THE END

www.ingramcontent.com/pod-product-compliance
Lightning Source LLC
Chambersburg PA
CBHW061547250726
48657CB00006B/2345